D0726341

THE NHS: THINGS THAT NEED TO BE SAID

THE NHS: THINGS THAT NEED TO BE SAID

IAIN DALE

LEADING BRITAIN'S CONVERSATION
DAB DIGITAL RADIO | 97.3 FM

This book is loosely based on a lecture I gave
at Queen's Hospital, Romford in January 2014,
for the Leslie Oliver Oration.

In memory of Andy Wilson

First published 2015 by
Elliott and Thompson Limited
27 John Street
London WC1N 2BX
www.eandtbooks.com

ISBN: 978-1-78396-078-1

A catalogue record for this book is available from the
British Library.

Managing Editor, LBC: James Rea
Deputy Managing Editor, LBC: Tom Cheal

Typesetting: Marie Doherty
Printed in the UK by TJ International Ltd

global

Contents

Introduction   vii

1   Politics and the NHS   1
2   Private sector v. public sector   9
3   Targets, outcomes and a seven-day-a-week NHS   17
4   What is 'national' about the National Health Service?   27
5   The coming funding gap   35
6   Care and the patient experience   45
7   The challenges of population growth and demographic change   53
8   The challenges of personal responsibility   61
9   Still the NHS Cinderella: mental health   75
10   Transparency and the right to know   81
11   Diet and the nanny state   85

Conclusion   91
50 things which could make the NHS better   95

Introduction

Writing a short polemical book about the NHS when, inevitably, the readers of the book are bound to know far more about the subject than I do, is perhaps not the wisest thing for a political pundit and broadcaster to do.

Let me explain why I am writing this book. Each and every one of us uses the NHS. We have shared experiences, both good and bad. We all have opinions about what the NHS does well and what it doesn't do so well. My motivation is not to write a book which contains all the answers to the NHS's problems. That would be both stupid and impossible. Instead, it is to highlight some issues which are of concern to NHS users, the people who work in the NHS and those tasked with running it.

Any government wanting to get the best out of the NHS starts from a position where they know the NHS has huge amounts of public support. An Ipsos MORI poll in July 2014 found that more than half (52 per cent) of the public say the NHS is what makes them most proud to be British, placing it above the armed forces (47 per cent), the royal family (33 per cent), Team GB (26 per cent) and the BBC (22 per cent). Despite recent coverage of care failings and the increasing financial squeeze, we are prouder of the health service than we were two years ago, shortly after the Olympics (52 per cent now compared with 45 per cent then).

Furthermore, according to the Ipsos MORI Global Trends Survey, Britain is the second most positive country, out of nineteen, surveyed about the quality of their healthcare, with only Belgium rating their healthcare more highly. But . . . And here's a very big BUT. The same survey found only one in ten of us (9 per cent) say that we expect quality to improve over the coming years, while 43 per cent think it will get worse. This makes us among the least optimistic of the twenty countries surveyed, and reflects concerns about the sustainability of the NHS in the future.

So that's the context.

What I am going to attempt to do is identify some issues which I think will dominate the health agenda over the next decade. I want to challenge orthodox NHS thinking and say a few things which I think need to be said, but don't always seem to form part of the current debate. And forgive me if I use a couple of personal experiences to illustrate some of the points I want to make.

In many ways, senior health professionals and those in government and opposition have much in common — even if that thought might fill the latter with a degree of horror.

The government is trying to wrestle with the demands of an empowered, knowledgeable twenty-first-century consumer base while NHS staff are all operating within a structure designed for a mid-twentieth-century command control system of healthcare provision.

There is another communality of interest — NHS staff all have a fair idea of what needs to be done, but no one in politics is courageous enough to articulate either the problems or the solutions. And, sadly, I do not see that changing either under any government we might have in the foreseeable future. No one is prepared to think the unthinkable, say the unsayable, much less implement the doable.

1
Politics and the NHS

Politicians treat the NHS as a political football, insisting on initiative after initiative, to prove that there really is ACTION THIS DAY, and yet consistently fail to plan for the long term. They seem to think that structural reform and targets will yield results — and sometimes, in the short term, they do, but who can really say that they can think of a single health secretary who has been able to plan for the long term — of either party? During the thirteen years of the last Labour government there were six different health secretaries.

The Conservatives under Margaret Thatcher and John Major did a little better and managed only seven in eighteen years. The coalition government has had two different health secretaries. So a health secretary serves for an average of a little over two years. Of the fifteen holders of this post since 1979, very few had any direct experience of health policy before they took on the job. So they spend six months reading themselves into the job and the last six months trying to save themselves from being sacked. This gives them each just a year to make an impact. A few years ago, the Adam Smith Institute published a report which opened that:

> Secretaries of state and their junior ministers come and go with sometimes breath-taking frequency. But the one thing they all have in common is the desire to make headline-grabbing changes to advance their careers. As a result the NHS is besieged by a bewildering array of initiatives from one minister, only for him or her to be replaced by another minister with their own (often conflicting) ideas. Politicians tend to think that they can improve the health service by simply giving orders, or setting targets. But such measures always have perverse effects, distorting clinical priorities and encouraging creative accounting. NHS policy should be determined by medical priorities and not by political ones.

Bearing in mind that the NHS is one of the world's largest organisations, this way of running it is utter madness. If IBM or Glaxo changed their chief executive every two years, their share prices would plummet and within a short time the company would be considered a basket case.

And so we constantly hear pleas to take the politics out of the NHS. Liam Fox, when he was Shadow Health Secretary, said it. Various Labour ministers have said it. Andrew Lansley said it. Jeremy Hunt actually believes it. But surely none of them can be so naive. Well, it seems the general public agree with them. A poll for the British Medical Association conducted by Ipsos MORI found two-thirds of the general public wanted the NHS to manage itself without the involvement of politicians. Another 46 per cent also said politicians should have low or no involvement in how the NHS is run. They are all wrong. We have to have democratic accountability in the NHS.

After all, the fact that the Health Service eats up £115 billion — a sixth (!) of public expenditure — means that the way that money is spent has to be made accountable, and that has to be through the political system. The trouble is that half of this sum has, according to the Wanless Report, gone on price inflation and extra pay — 25 per cent to consultants and 23 per cent to GPs.

Was that the right thing to do? Voters will be judge and jury on that point. It had to be a political decision, not one made by a faceless independent board. So any politician who calls for politics to be taken out of the NHS is likely to be doing it to get a cheap round of applause on *Question Time* and can safely be ignored. It isn't going to happen, and nor should it.

That's my view but, interestingly, the think-tank the Adam Smith Institute (ASI) begs to differ. Its briefing paper documents the bewildering and counterproductive range of political initiatives and interference which, it says, has wreaked havoc on our nation's healthcare system.

The paper's proposal is for a distinguished panel of health professionals to be appointed to run the NHS, to allocate its budget, determine its priorities, and operate it according to medical needs rather than political aims. A YouGov poll taken on the subject showed massive popular support for precisely such a proposal, with 69 per cent in favour and only 12 per cent against.

The NHS budget would be set by Parliament every five years, and increased each year in line with inflation. The ASI's YouGov poll showed that this idea, too, enjoys widespread popular support, with 74 per cent in favour. The suggestion that 'the NHS has become a political football' receives 72 per cent backing.

Whatever the merits of the ASI's proposals or those of the Conservatives, an independent NHS certainly isn't going to happen when we have such consummate political brains in Number 10. Think back to the Gordon Brown government.

I'm told that the Deep Clean initiative wasn't thought up in the Department of Health. It came direct from the Number 10 Policy Unit, who gave the Department of Health a few hours in which to consider how to make it work. It was duly announced by the prime minister, who made it sound as if this would be the only measure needed to eradicate MRSA and C. difficile from our hospitals. Indeed, when I heard about it, I too thought it sounded a deeply sensible measure.

That is until I switched on a radio phone-in and heard a succession of health service professionals slam it. Not a single one of them thought it would work. Not a single one of them was taken in by it. It was at that point I started to wonder if this gargantuan political brain was actually as formidable as we'd all been led to believe and that his administration wasn't just as driven by spin as the previous one.

Just as a transport secretary is judged on whether their tenure of office is free of a major rail crash or transport disaster, a health secretary is now judged on whether he or she can keep NHS stories off the front pages. That's why Andrew Lansley had to go, and was replaced by a politician with a far better bedside manner.

So that's my first thing which needs to be said: you can't take politics out of the NHS, and nor should you. In fact, as I shall explain later, I think we ought to be having a big debate about the NHS, but we are being denied that debate because whenever any politician on the right or left, but mainly the right, has the temerity to criticise the NHS, he or she is jumped on and warned about the consequences of having a go at a beloved institution.

If you point out that outcomes in the NHS are in most areas way below other comparable nations, you are accused of denigrating people who work so hard in the NHS or advocating privatisation even when you're not. If the NHS can't stand up to robust critique, it says an awful lot about the arguments of its very vocal defenders.

2
Private sector
v. public sector

The private sector versus public sector debate has bedevilled health policy for some time. It lies at the very core of the failure of politicians to provide the leadership the NHS needs.

The public good, private bad mindset which is held by many politicians on the left is equally matched by the private good, public bad attitudes often prevalent on the right. Only in this country could this happen. Even in these days of supposed consensus, these attitudes still prevail.

Do any of these politicians think people care if they are treated privately or in an NHS hospital, if they get the treatment they want, where they want, when they want it? Of course not. Yet people who use BUPA or other private health providers are made to feel as if they are somehow being elitist, rather than being praised for taking responsibility for their own healthcare and not burdening the NHS with their demands. A ComRes poll in July 2014 showed that two in three people (67 per cent) say that they do not mind if health services are provided by a private company or the NHS as long as they remain free of charge.

Beveridge and Bevan never meant for the NHS to have to meet every single demand ever made of it. Two systems can work happily together as long as each respects the other. For too long in this country Labour politicians have seen private medicine as a class enemy and Tory politicians have viewed the NHS as something for other people to use, not them.

David Cameron makes great play out of the fact that he is a regular user of the NHS. He had a disabled son whose fits made regular overnight stays in a local hospital a normal occurrence for him. His view was shaped by his experience. He put the NHS at the top of his agenda. He says his three priorities can be summed up in three letters: N. H. S.

One of Cameron's first acts was to abolish the Tory policy of encouraging private sector health-care. George Osborne said in opposition: 'We are having no truck with ideas for some alternative funding mechanism like social insurance.

Nor are we looking to help fund escape routes from public services for the few who can afford it, which is why we have moved away from the idea of the patients' passport.'

All very well, but where are we going to get the extra capacity the NHS needs, if the private sector is not embraced in a way it hasn't been before? Ministers in the last Labour government would freely admit they would not have been able to reduce waiting lists without utilising private sector capacity.

Let's not pretend that private sector involvement in the provision of healthcare is anything new. Most people use private sector dentists. GPs are effectively in the private sector, as are most osteopaths and physiotherapists. A lot of primary care is provided by the private sector — the out of hours service and 111 to name but two examples.

Drugs are provided by private sector suppliers. Chemists and dispensaries have never been in the public sector and no one has ever suggested they should be. It was recently reported with some horror in the *Guardian* that

70 per cent of NHS contracts are with the private sector. They put this down to the Lansley reforms, omitting to say that the private sector has always played a major role in health provision.

Opponents of the private sector also raise the spectre of the NHS introducing charges, conveniently forgetting that patients already pay prescription charges. From time to time, the issues of charging for hospital food or GP visits are floated, but quickly ditched until the howl of public outrage subsides.

However, on radio phone-ins such as my own, the idea of charging for NHS services is quite popular in some areas. For example, people ask why the taxpayer should pay for the treatment of people who bring their own misfortune on themselves.

People who binge drink on a Friday night often end up in A&E. Why shouldn't they be charged? People who regret getting a tattoo can apparently have it removed courtesy of the NHS. But where do you draw the line? Charge smokers for lung cancer treatment? Charge obese people for diabetes drugs? Another one for the too difficult box, I suspect.

Very few people have anything nice to say about NICE, the National Institute for Health and Care Excellence. And let me be no exception.

It was set up by the Labour government with the best of intentions. Part of its mission was to end the variation in medical treatment across the country and ensure that if a drug was found to be effective, patients should not have to fight to get it. Clearly there needs to be a body which licenses drugs, but there is a huge suspicion that too many drugs are still licensed through budgetary consideration rather than clinical need.

And, in turn, drugs which are available in some parts of the country are not in others — for much the same reason. And if a cancer patient should have the temerity to decide to use their life savings to fund their treatment using a drug which for budgetary reasons is not available via the NHS, what does the NHS do?

Instead of saying 'thank you very much for helping us out and paying for your own drugs', it refuses to continue any treatment for that patient. See? Public good, private bad. It's the politics of socialist envy and basically says that just because everyone can't have it, you can't either. So people die. Is that really what should be happening? I don't think so. It's an exemplification of the kind of dogma which has bedevilled our public-sector thinking over many decades.

This is what happened to one of my listeners who emailed me her story:

'My twenty-three-year-old son has just been turned down for a course of drugs for his acute vasculitis, which he has been waiting around five months for. It costs around £4,000 for the course. His consultant has stated that it's one of the few drugs that would really make a difference. He had to go back into hospital in the early hours of Tuesday morning, and they have probably spent half that amount, running more tests, and keeping him in under observation, when he could have been back at work, earning a living, paying taxes, and with a reasonably pain-free outcome. How short-sighted can you be?'

Well, it's a good question, isn't it? I am surprised that no one has yet taken the NHS, or NICE, to the European Court of Human Rights over issues like this. I suspect it is a matter of time. Perhaps then the postcode lottery may forcibly be brought to an end.

No other country's health system operates in such a bigoted and uncaring way. The sooner we eradicate this sort of thinking, the better. If we are to get anywhere in improving standards of healthcare and quality of outcomes, then surely it is obvious that the public and private sector healthcare systems need to operate side by side and help each other where possible.

3
Targets, outcomes and a seven-day-a-week NHS

People questioned whether the Conservatives would also embrace the target-driven culture which so obsessed the previous Labour government. It seemed to be the only way to increase throughput, although NHS managers continue to try to convince us that we can do with fewer and fewer beds and various management consultants still try to hypnotise us into really believing their reports that people prefer to be treated at home, no matter what their affliction.

The Conservatives professed to want to abolish the target culture, yet have so far failed to explain how this can improve capacity. Because the truth is that weakening targets has led to capacity issues in many areas of the NHS.

Labour brought in targets, at least in part, to improve outcomes. They, like many others, were mystified by the fact that despite investing ever more money, other countries did consistently better than us in terms of outcomes.

Take cancer. For years Britain has outspent many other countries in cancer research and treatment, yet our survivability record is shockingly poor. The Organisation for Economic Cooperation and Development (OECD) brands it 'unacceptable' and it is easy to see why. In 2013 the OECD reported that women with breast cancer were more likely to reach the five-year survival point in almost all countries other than Britain, with only the Czech Republic, Poland and Ireland trailing behind. Only the Czech Republic, Poland and Denmark had worse rates for surviving bowel cancer than Britain while cervical cancer rates were worse in only Poland and Ireland. This ought to be a source of national embarrassment, but we are constantly told that we have the best health service in the world.

Part of the reason for this lamentable performance in cancer survivability is our chronic lack of funding for life-saving cancer drugs. Drugs which are freely available in most other developed countries are simply not on the NICE list. The government promised to alleviate this disastrous policy by creating the Cancer Drugs Fund, but this has been fought every step of the way by NHS managers, who for reasons best known to themselves don't want to see these drugs made available to the very people who need them most. Furthermore, they have also restricted the availability of advanced radiotherapy so that pathetically few patients ever benefit from it. Meanwhile, the very machines used for this sit unused because NHS England refuses to provide funding for various cancer treatments.

Former England rugby captain Lawrence Dallaglio had been tasked by the health secretary, Jeremy Hunt, to help devise the implementation of the Cancer Drugs Fund following the death of his mother from cancer. It appears he has been thwarted every step of the way by the travails of NHS bureaucracy. And, meanwhile, cancer patients in this country continue to die more quickly than they would otherwise have done.

Figures quoted in the *Sunday Times* in July reveal that the number of patients being offered advanced radiotherapy treatment is actually falling. Since NHS England took control of the issue in April 2013, ten per cent fewer people

are being treated. The number given the trans-
formative SABR treatment on rare and complex
cancers have plummeted by 70 per cent in little over a year. The Lib Dem MP Tessa Munt,
whose Freedom of Information request elicited
the figures said: 'NHS England is simply letting
patients die'. Campaigners wonder what agenda
is driving NHS England's policy. Last year they
agreed to spend £5 million a year — peanuts in
a budget of £120 billion — to conduct clinical
trials on spine, liver and pelvis cancers and
ensure advanced radiotherapy was available
throughout the country. They have now reneged
on that. They now say they won't back clinical
trials, they will only help half the number of
patients previously agreed, they won't start it
until April 2015 and there is no money to fund
anything else.

This is but one example of where NHS
bureaucracy and false priorities are affect-
ing patient care for the worse. There are many
more. And the thing is, nothing will change
unless an iron fist at the centre grips the issue.

If the new chief executive of NHS England thinks that employing fifty new highly paid managers is more important than improving cancer survivability then, Houston, we really do have a problem. Lawrence Dallaglio sums it up in an interview with the *Sunday Times* on 6 July 2014:

> 'England should be a leader rather than a follower in the way we treat cancer. We are languishing way down the bottom of the table. It's embarrassing. It would appear it's not because we don't have the necessary resource. It's down to bureaucracy as far as I can see. This needs to be resolved now, not next year or in another four years. It angers me and I'm sure it angers everyone.'

Quite.

Some think the biggest problem in the area of cancer survivability is the continuing blight of late referrals by GPs. But is naming and shaming badly performing GPs really the answer to this? Won't it just mean that to cover themselves GPs will refer everyone?

Outcomes are also adversely affected by the fact that the NHS seems to operate on a five-day-a-week basis, rather than seven.

One thing I noticed when my mother spent three awful weeks in hospital (more of that in chapter six), was that the place more or less shut down at weekends, as do GP surgeries in large part. How odd. Are people not supposed to get ill at weekends? Why is it that operating theatres are mostly empty at weekends? Surely we should be moving towards a seven-day NHS, with equality of service provision throughout those seven days?

If we are to get better outcomes, surely that has to happen over time? It comes back to the point I made earlier about twenty-first-century medicine operating within the straitjacket of a 1940s system. Why is it that GP surgeries offer appointments at times the majority of the population isn't available to go to them? Why aren't there more evening and weekend appointment slots? I run a publishing company and I reckon I lose hundreds of man hours of work a year as my employees say, 'Oh, I have got a doctor's appointment', as if that is a reason why they should be allowed time off to the detriment of the company. That may sound harsh, but multiply that all over the economy and we're all losing out just because GPs have always worked that way and seem immune to the changes of a modern-day economy.

I don't blame GPs for negotiating the GP contract back in 2004 which allowed their pay to rocket despite opting out of providing out-of-hours cover. Who wouldn't? Quite what the then health secretary Alan Milburn was thinking of, God alone knows, and it is this government which has been left the legacy.

And that legacy, at least in part, is A&E departments which are bursting at the seams with patients who shouldn't even be there. We now have the frankly ludicrous scenario of A&E departments employing GPs to see all the people who visit A&E departments because they have no way of seeing their GP at weekends — or at least, that is their perception. Admittedly this started back in the 1990s, but the practice has grown exponentially in recent times. These GPs are employed for one reason, and one reason only — to allow the A&Es to meet their waiting-time targets.

4
What is 'national' about the National Health Service?

Before the last election the then leading Lib Dem politician Chris Huhne said — rather courageously, I thought — that the NHS needed to be broken up into local units. Quite what he meant by local, he didn't say, but everyone knows that turning round the NHS is like turning round an oil tanker.

It takes years, sometimes decades, for structural and organisational changes to come into effect. And by the time you've worked out whether they were right in the first place, it is too late or priorities have changed.

So we've had various forms of local accountability over the past twenty years, none of which have proved satisfactory. In theory, the smaller versions of Primary Care Trusts ought to have provided that, but were often so saddled with debt that they could not respond to local needs. They therefore had to embark on a rationalisation process which local people just could not buy into. They felt they were being hoodwinked, that elaborate consultation exercises were generally a sham and that the decision had already been made. I saw this at first-hand in north Norfolk, where I was a candidate at the 2005 election.

People kept being told that everything was done in their best interests, but they just didn't believe it. It even got to the point where people were even less likely to believe the words of a Health Trust official than those of a politician. People just didn't buy the argument that community hospitals had to close and that the same level of care could be provided in people's own homes.

They couldn't see why a local dementia care unit had to be shut, only ten years after it had been built specifically for that purpose. Local people weren't convinced and local politicians weren't convinced either. And, even if they had been, could they, could I, as one of them, have had the courage to say so?

This culminated in the ridiculous sight of Labour Party Chairman Hazel Blears joining a protest in her constituency against the closure of a maternity unit her own government wanted to shut.

What had brought this about? Was it *really* all about medical advances meaning that maternity care needed to be concentrated in one place, or that community hospitals were no longer relevant due to the level of care being provided at major hospitals?

Or was it more a question of funding, and the NHS was being forced to cut its cloth according to its funding? Most people suspect that many of the closures are being forced by the latter rather than the former — and this despite health funding having more than doubled since 1997.

People are, rightly, asking where the money has gone. They blame politicians, but they also blame so-called NHS bureaucrats who seem happy to accept a situation where a hospital has more managers than beds, more managers than nurses. They see an organisation which is top-heavy with middle management and a cadre of politicians who seem powerless or lack the will to do anything about it. And the thing is, in this ever less deferential society, people simply will not sit there and be told that others know what's best for them.

On another level, GPs see it every day in their surgeries. Patients engage in self-diagnosis at a level previously undreamed of. They look at the Internet and wonder why, if a drug is available in Texas, they can't be prescribed it locally at their surgery. Some patients even turn up with their laptops to explain to their doctor how they have arrived at a particular conclusion. Now doctors realise what politicians have had to put up with for decades!

I wonder whether the NHS can continue as a truly National Health Service. But let's be honest. We're deluding ourselves if we truly believe it is even now, a NATIONAL health service. Scotland and Wales run their own NHSs. And the English NHS contains such wide variations that it can't be said to be truly national.

Treatments that are available in one area, are not in another. Outcomes vary so widely that the use of the word national becomes laughable, if not redundant.

For instance, there's no national policy on visitor parking at hospitals. In some areas it is free, in others it costs up to £500 a week. What's 'national' about that? I think there's something immoral about charging someone to visit a family member who is ill in hospital, yet we have to recognise that car parks cost money to maintain. A Conservative MP, Robert Halfon, has launched a campaign to persuade the Health Secretary to abolish all parking charges throughout England. This would cost £200 million a year in lost revenue. Quite how you would then stop the facility being abused isn't yet clear, but Halfon argue the cost could be recouped through the use of generic rather than branded drugs. Maybe, but if it were that simple, why hasn't it been done before? But there's no doubt that any health secretary who abolished hospital parking charges, or even reduced them, would be seen as a bit of a national hero.

So why don't we ditch the sentiment about a 'national' health service and recognise that the costs of running a national institution may sometimes outweigh any benefits there are. The main benefit ought to be the massive purchasing power that such an organisation enjoys, but we all know that NHS procurement procedures are a joke, and almost as inefficient and incompetent as those in the Ministry of Defence — and that's saying something. Suppliers and drugs companies run rings around NHS purchasing managers and get away with imposing what is laughably called 'NHS inflation'. So let's stop pretending. About the only benefit of primary care trusts was that they didn't pretend at all. They were proof positive that everything is local.

I've mentioned the postcode lottery before but, in effect, you can't really avoid having different standards in different areas if you believe in localism. How do you have more local decision-taking and less centralised control without some degree of regional variation? The question is, how much variation is the patient willing to put up with?

5
The coming funding gap

Funding dilemmas permeate all areas of the NHS. A huge amount of money has been channelled into the NHS in recent years, but it's not just politicians who are failing to see an outcome — it's patients. Even though nearly half of it has gone on meeting inflation and pay increases, a doubling of financial input ought to have led to a double-figure rise in productivity.

It has not and people want to know why. There will soon be a funding shortfall of £30 billion. How can this be? Is it a problem of acute financial mismanagement? Is health service inflation really so high? Why are efficiency savings so hard to make?

The Wanless Report rightly highlighted a real fear that if the NHS does not prove it can use its money better, taxpayers will no longer be willing to cough up for it.

This is perhaps unnecessarily apocalyptic, but it is something which politicians would do well to take note of. We are already seeing this in the area of constitutional issues, Europe and the devolution settlement; if voters think they are being taken for granted they react accordingly.

Currently, we spend more than £115 billion on the NHS, almost one-sixth of every pound the government spends on behalf of the taxpayer. And yet every day we read that more needs to be spent if the NHS isn't to collapse within the next five years. Vested interest after vested interest puts its case for an increase in funding, imagining that all these extra pounds will be picked off the taxpayer money tree and magically appear to fund whatever is on their latest wish list. They point out that if we didn't renew Trident, for example, an extra £100 billion would be available to fund the NHS. If we hadn't invaded Iraq, another £20 billion would have been free for the NHS to use. These arguments are as facile as they are ridiculous. In theory we could spend our entire public expenditure on the NHS and still there would be some who would say the government should borrow more. In the end, politicians are there to make choices.

A political party outlines its manifesto at

an election and then says how it is going to be paid for. That's the theory, anyway. At the next election, all parties ought to explain their spending plans on the NHS. At the last election the Conservatives promised to ring-fence the NHS budget and increase it in real terms each year. This they have done, albeit by only 0.1 per cent. Commentators point out that this means there have still been real-terms cuts because health service inflation is still rampant and the demands made on the NHS by an increasingly elderly population are ever greater. They are right, but does that mean we have to accede to requests to grow funding by up to 5 per cent in real terms each year, bearing in mind that in cash terms that means an extra £5—7 billion on top of inflation, equivalent to an income tax rise of two or three pence?

Having said that, a ComRes poll in July 2014 showed that in theory people would be willing to contribute more. Asked if they would be prepared to pay more tax to maintain the current level of care and services provided by the NHS, 57 per cent agreed and 41 per cent disagreed.

The finding will encourage the Labour Party, which is considering an earmarked 'Health Tax' to help head off the looming NHS funding crisis.

An Ipsos MORI poll found that two-thirds of the public (65 per cent) favour increased funding to maintain current service provision while only 14 per cent think that services should be limited in order to stay within the present budget. The majority (79 per cent) want the NHS protected from any spending cuts — a higher proportion than for schools (51 per cent), care for the elderly (51 per cent) or the police (39 per cent).

No, the NHS needs to cut its cloth just like the rest of the economy. The funding gap will be bridged in one of three ways: the NHS needs reduce its costs, increase its revenue or restrict what it does. I suggest it should do all three. But how?

First of all, it needs to improve its procurement procedures. It is one of the biggest purchasers of goods and services in the country, yet there are huge suspicions that it doesn't use its buying power aggressively enough. Maybe the

NHS could learn something from its local government colleagues.

The NHS is by far the biggest purchaser of drugs in the country, yet too often it buys the expensive brand names rather than generic alternatives, which are a fraction of the cost. It employs far too many managers and administrators whose functions are far removed from the provision of health services. There are far too many PR and communications people, too many bloated human resources departments. I could go on. No one is saying you can run a hospital without managers, but too much of NHS trust management and hospital management is now concerned with 'back covering' rather than the provision of proper medical care.

Something also needs to be done about the astonishing number of people in the NHS who trouser high six-figure salaries. Don't get me wrong, high-achieving people deserve to earn a good salary, but can anyone seriously justify a hospital chief executive earning double what the prime minister does? Or, in some cases, treble?

Take the Medway Foundation Hospital where thirty managers earn more than £100,000. That's just administrators, and doesn't include consultants or surgeons. This is in a hospital which itself says it needs to employ 120 more nurses. In 2014 the chairman earned £200,000 for a two-day week. Nice work if you can get it. Its chief executive earned £360,000 for a four-day week. Its so-called treasurer received a whopping £540,000 a year. The chairman was also entitled to claim £17,000 a year in expenses with no need to provide proof of how the money was spent.

You can bet that if it's happening in Medway, it is being repeated all over the country. When the Mid Staffordshire NHS Foundation Trust went into administration, eighty-five of its employees were on a six-figure salary, up from seventy-four the year before. The finance director who presided over its financial meltdown was earning £340,000 a year.

And, of course, there have been various scandals about six-figure pay-offs to highly paid staff who have failed in their job, but then sometimes, only months later, reappear in a senior position in another hospital or NHS Trust.

Why is there so little public outrage about all this? Even the chief executive of the NHS 'only' earns £189,000 a year. I regard that as a fair salary for someone doing that job. But how then, can an individual hospital chief executive rake in more than double that? According to the *Guardian*, in 2013 there were forty-eight administrators in the NHS who earned more than the prime minister (£142,000) and 291 who earned more than £100,000. That is one in twenty of NHS England's 6,115 managerial staff. This didn't include hospital staff. The average pay level of hospital administrators was more than £75,000, far higher than in any other part of the public sector. In the whole of the NHS there were 7,800 people who earned more than £100,000.

It's the same among GPs. Following the renegotiation of their contracts in 2004, their pay has rocketed. Official figures show that 16,000

GPs are now earning more than £100,000 and 600 are earning more than £200,000. Ten years ago, only 4,000 GPs earned such sums. GPs have seen their average pay rocket by 41 per cent in the last ten years, while nurses have seen their pay rise by a more steady 18 per cent. The number of patients each GP cares for has fallen by 11 per cent, and the number of doctors has risen by 23 per cent. And yet still the BMA GPs' committee reckons their members are hard done by. The proof seems to point to the exact opposite.

Most defenders of the existing status quo in the NHS will react with horror whenever the words 'income' or 'revenue' are mentioned. But let's not ignore the fact that the NHS isn't always free at the point of use. Dare I mention dentistry? And many people in England pay for prescriptions, let us not forget.

There are ways of generating revenue without damaging the founding tenets of the NHS. We could save several hundred million pounds a year by charging foreign visitors for using NHS facilities, for example. It has been suggested charging people £10 to visit a GP. Why not charge drunks every time they turn up in an A&E facility? Why should all diabetes patients get their prescriptions free of charge? Most Type 2 diabetes patients have brought their condition on themselves by their own bad diets. Believe me, I know. Operating theatres lie empty at weekends. Why not rent them out to the private sector?

There are also far too many quangos and regulators operating in the NHS, all with very highly paid leaders and executives. They should be culled. Not all of them, but at least a third, and the next government needs to set up a review into the effectiveness of each of them.

We also have to accept that when the NHS was set up, it was not designed to meet every demand made of it. It was certainly not set up to provide cosmetic surgery on the taxpayer. Despite what the purists may have you believe, we already restrict some treatments — dentistry and physiotherapy being two examples — so perhaps we need to have a national debate on whether that list should be expanded.

6
Care and the patient experience

We all make judgements on the NHS depend-
ing on whether we work for it, we are patients
ourselves or we have family or friends who use
it. All our judgements are based on our own
experience or that of those close to us. Indeed,
doctors, surgeons and nurses are not immune to
this, with surveys showing that in some hospitals 70 per cent of those who work there wouldn't
want their family members to be treated in their
own hospitals.

It's all anecdotal evidence, but that's the only
evidence an individual has got. So when learned
academic studies are published that are at vari-
ance with our own experience, we tend to speak
out. Clearly, people always tend to highlight
the negative rather than the positive, which is
why whenever I host a phone-in on my radio
show about a particular aspect of the NHS, I am
always careful to solicit positive as well as negative callers.

Ann Clwyd, the Labour MP, became a bit of
a bête noir for some in the medical profession
when she told of the terrible care her husband

had received courtesy of a hospital in Cardiff. He died. She made a tearful speech telling of their experience and was later asked by David Cameron to head a review looking into complaints against the NHS.

Her report made very sad reading for all concerned with the standards of nursing care in this country. I regret to say it chimed with me, for my mother went through a terrible experience at Addenbrookes Hospital in Cambridge, after which she sadly died. It was a horrible experience for her, for my father, for my sisters and myself. Throughout it all, we felt powerless. It turns out that she was put on the Liverpool Care pathway. We were never told about it. No one seemed to be able to tell us what was happening to her.

She was put on the wrong drugs. She kept telling us 'they're trying to kill me'. We put it down to the effects of the drugs but, in the end, perhaps she was trying to tell us something that we were too deaf to hear. We put our trust in the hospital and they let us down. More importantly, they let her down.

The standard of nursing care was lamentable. There were different nurses every day. I reckon she had a hundred different nurses in the three weeks she was in that ward. I'd love anyone to tell me how there can be any continuity of care in such circumstances.

I queried why, whenever I visited, there was never a nurse that I recognised. 'Oh, it's the forty-eight hour week that's to blame,' one said. 'And we get put on different wards each day.'

Half of them seemed to be agency nurses, some with a variable grasp of English — never a good thing when dealing with older patients. They kept trying to feed her totally inappropriate food, when a cursory look at her notes would have told them it was wrong.

She was left, sometimes for hours, in soiled sheets. In the end, my two sisters and I operated a shift system because we couldn't let her be alone. We ignored the visiting hours, and the nurses allowed us to because it took work away from them. And the thing is, it wasn't because there weren't enough of them. There were.

When we eventually realised that my mother was going to die, we decided to take her home. The thought of her dying in that place was too awful for us to contemplate. But even then they were so incompetent that I was forced to book a private ambulance to take her home because the NHS ambulance consistently didn't turn up.

She spent two weeks at home, and it was here that the NHS came up trumps with her wonderful GP visiting at least twice a day and providing just the support that she, and we, her carers, needed. I shall never forget what that wonderful GP did that week.

My mother died at home looking out on the garden she loved, surrounded by her family.

I should have made an official complaint about Addenbrookes. I should have raised merry hell with the hospital bosses and, you know what, I am ashamed that I didn't. I just couldn't bear the thought of reliving it all. I let my mother down, and I let all those who followed her down. While she was lying in there, unable to do anything for herself, I kept thinking about other patients who had no family to care for them. We were in a position to do things, but there are many older people whose families can't or won't support them in the way we could.

It was only when I read about Ann Clwyd's experience that I actually did something about it. She had thousands of letters and emails from people who had gone through the same thing.

Blame is easy to ascribe, but it is often misplaced. I have thought long and hard about how these things are allowed to happen. In truth there is no one single person or group of people who are to blame. And, let's face it, blame rarely gets us anywhere. But there are clearly questions to be asked about current standards of nursing care in some of our hospitals.

So when I heard Jeremy Hunt say, almost on his first day in the job as health secretary, that he was concerned about the fact that nursing care was becoming increasingly depersonalised, my ears pricked up. But when he suggested that nurses should do a year's on-the-job training before embarking on degrees, he was met with a hailstorm of abuse from the usual vested interests. 'A really stupid idea,' said the RCN. A truly pathetic response, which one might expect from a trade union but not from a Royal College — the very same Royal College which failed to spot any problems at the Mid Staffs hospital.

It seems to me that aspects of nursing training are not fit for purpose. Jeremy Hunt said this 'culture of defensiveness' must cease and doctors and nurses must 'say sorry' when things go wrong in the NHS. Administrators blanch at that, saying, 'think of the legal consequences', but surely he's right. Indeed, there is now legal precedent that 'saying sorry' is not a legal admission of guilt.

Of course things will go wrong. In any organisation the size of the NHS, and with the risks involved in most medical procedures, there will always be mistakes and things will always go wrong on occasion. The challenge for the NHS is to find a way of acknowledging this in a way which doesn't undermine the whole system.

I think we also need to look at who we are recruiting into the nursing profession. It seems to be ridiculous that all nurses are now expected to have degrees or the equivalent. Surely we need a mix of abilities and aptitudes. Where are the good working-class girls who used to be the backbone of the nursing profession? They may not have had an O level between them, but they knew all about providing fantastic care. They weren't too proud to do the dirtier jobs that some nurses seem to think it isn't their job to do nowadays. I don't know what proportion of nurses in the NHS come from other countries, but how rigorously do we check their backgrounds and qualifications — or even linguistic abilities? The NHS would collapse without foreign nurses and doctors, but I have always been slightly queasy about overtly recruiting them from countries which frankly are so poor that the best form of international aid we could offer them is not to steal their most capable medical staff.

7
The challenges of population growth and demographic change

One of the reasons the NHS has required an ever-growing budget is to cope with the challenges of population growth and demographic change. Over the next couple of decades the population will grow by ten million, in large part to immigration but also due to a higher birth rate among many immigrant communities.

The planning for that should already be underway, but I wonder if it is. Coupled with the added burden of an ever-growing older population, it is no wonder that the NHS is already creaking at the seams. But how far can the taxpayer's patience be stretched?

In addition, the pressures of an ageing population mean that the social care system is already creaking. We already spend one-sixth of our public spending on the NHS. If that proportion is to increase beyond a sixth, some incredibly difficult decisions will have to be taken elsewhere. But what should it rise to? It's a question even the new NHS Action Party can't or won't answer. Why not? A fifth? A quarter?

At some point decisions will have to be made about a) the scope of treatments b) restricting the scope of NHS functions and c) cutting ever-burgeoning costs.

I don't know how many planners there are in the NHS or how much they are paid, but it's a safe bet to guess that however many there are, they are very highly paid. But for what? Because they do seem to get things spectacularly wrong. Why, for example, when a decade ago there were 2,500 more GPs than hospital doctors, there are now 38,200 hospital doctors compared to 31,700 GPs? And this at a time when government policy is to treat people in their homes or communities rather than in hospital. Surely a decade ago the planners and bureaucrats should have been able to predict that more GPs would be needed, rather than hospital doctors?

Even worse than that, we continue to train doctors in areas where we already have enough of them. As Sarah Wollaston, a former GP herself, and now chair of the Health Select Committee says:

'We've got the wrong workforce. What we do, still, is train too many doctors out of medical school, to become acute hospital specialists in specialities for which there are no jobs. They might have four or five years training to become a particular hospital specialist when everybody knows there won't be a job for all of them. And in general practice we've got huge vacancies.'

There are many areas where the NHS is said to be in crisis, but general practice is certainly about to be one of them if present trends continue. Much of it stems back to 2004 and the contract signed by the then health secretary Alan Milburn and GPs about their hours of service and pay. He was warned at the time that removing GPs' out of hours obligations and, despite this, giving them huge amounts more money would prove to be a disaster, but he went ahead anyway. And we are now reaping the whirlwind that followed.

People complain they can't get appointments when they want them and that at weekends it's almost impossible. It's not all down to that contract, but also because not enough GPs have been recruited. Population growth on its own — eminently foreseeable by NHS planners — should have set off warning sirens both in the minds of NHS managers and politicians, but it's only now, when patient approval of GP services is dropping like a stone, that people are waking up to the fact that a crisis is coming, and approaching very quickly.

What we have effectively got are the wrong skills, in the wrong workforce, in the wrong number, in the wrong place. If we were starting from scratch, we certainly wouldn't want to be in this position.

The problem is that you can't just switch on a tap and recruit several thousand more GPs just like that. They take years to train. There are also far too many barriers to former GPs looking to re-enter the workforce. For example, female GPs who have taken a decade out to have children face having to pay for their own retraining — this at a time when the health service is crying out for them to come back. Remember that phrase so beloved of Labour ministers, 'joined-up government'? There's obviously some way to go before it can apply to the NHS.

With a growing elderly population, how will we cope with the mounting demands on elderly care in hospitals and social care outside? The challenge for the government, and indeed NHS planners, is how to integrate the two. Otherwise we have to try to find bureaucratic ways of achieving a separation of health from social care in terms of costs and resources. There are far too many geriatric patients who take up bed space in hospitals because there is nowhere for them to be discharged to.

Successive governments have failed to plan for the future and although the coalition has announced a plan of action in this area, I wonder how many of us are convinced by it. Until politicians finally have the courage to tell people 'yes, you'll have to sell your home' to pay for social care, the debate will remain somewhat stagnant.

The state won't be able to meet every demand that is made of it in the area of social care and people should not be misled into thinking it ever will. Just look at the statistics. The number of people aged ninety or over has trebled in the last thirty years. The number of people who live to one hundred has gone up fivefold in the same period. Over the next twenty-five years the number of eighty-year-olds will double. The number of centenarians will rise from 13,000 at the moment to 111,000.

ONS projections say that increases in life-spans — attributed to improving medicine, growing wealth, healthier lifestyles and less physically demanding work — will lead to a society where more than one in five people is a pensioner. Think about that.

To the government's credit, they are reforming the pensions system to take into account these demographic changes, but where is the forward planning in the health and social care systems?

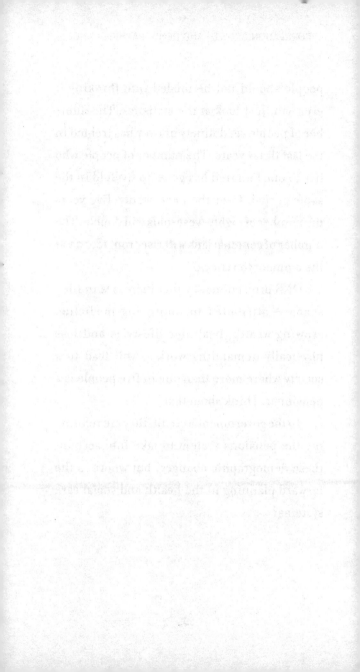

8
The challenges of personal responsibility

Personal responsibility is a phrase which seems to have largely gone out of fashion, not just in terms of our health, but in wider society too. If we all took responsibility for the food, drink and drugs we shovel into our bodies, it is not an unreasonable proposition to assert that the NHS would cost much less than it does. Successive governments have poured billions into educating us in how to look after our bodies and health, but huge numbers of us turn a complete blind eye. Even when we know what we eat, drink or smoke will damage our health and shorten our lives, we still do it. Have we really become so decadent that we think that we will all live forever no matter what damage we do to our bodies? Let's start with alcohol.

It was recently announced that NICE are launching a consultation on prescribing a new drug called Nalmefene which, according to the *Independent*, could help alcoholics quit drinking. Sorted! Well, not quite. The *Independent* headline screamed: 'Once-a-day pill to beat alcoholism gains backing from health officials'.

If only it were that simple. All the pill does, apparently, is help someone cut their alcohol consumption by up to 50 per cent. It is already prescribed in Scotland and has been available in the USA for at least ten years. Here comes the rub. If it were prescribed to all 600,000 people with alcohol dependency problems, it would cost the NHS an extra £600 million. But, just as important, it also erodes people's sense of personal responsibility. Counselling and help from groups like Alcoholics Anonymous may well bring far better results than a pill, which will inevitably be taken by those who don't feel they have the mental willpower to stop drinking altogether. Dr Des Spence, a GP in Glasgow, is not a fan of Nalmefene. He penned a piece for the *BMA Journal* in February criticising the decision by the NHS in Scotland to prescribe Nalmefene at a cost of £84 a month per patient. He was also very sceptical of the significance of the trial findings. 'Surely these resources would be better spent improving alcohol counselling services?' he wrote.

But if we are really serious about personal responsibility, we need to look at the growing problem of diabetes. This disease is already costing £10 billion a year to the NHS in prescription drugs and dealing with the effects of diabetes. By 2035, that figure will have risen to at least £17 billion. Diabetes will never be eradicated, but Type 2 diabetes is a disease that is easily preventable if people actually heed good dietary and exercise advice. And this is where I embarrass myself. Let me tell you the story of my Type 2 diabetes. Back in January 2008, I wrote this on my blog:

'I got a bit of bad news on Wednesday, when I was told I had been diagnosed with diabetes. It wasn't a shock as — using my enormous medical expertise :) — I had already diagnosed myself. For some time I have had an unquenchable thirst and other symptoms. Luckily it is Type 2, so I won't have to inject myself every day.

I went to see my doctor yesterday evening who told me that it 'could be a blessing in disguise'. I must admit I wondered about her sanity when she said that, but she may be right. To have it diagnosed at my age means I can beat it if I adopt the right diet and exercise routines and get my blood sugar levels down. This will 'unfur' arteries and lessen the risk of heart or kidney problems in the future.

So I guess I am going to be harvesting lots of info about diabetes from various websites over the next few weeks and learning from other people about their experiences. My father was diagnosed with it seven years ago and my godmother had it too. She had to inject herself twice a day and had been doing it since the 1960s. I am now going to have to take ten pills a day for the foreseeable future. Even worse, I won't be able to drink Lemon Lucozade any more!

I must admit I was rather shocked by the reaction of a couple of people I have told face-to-face. They seemed to equate it with being told that I had a terminal illness. I don't see it that way at all. I count myself very lucky. I've had forty-five years of being totally healthy. In the last few weeks, a good friend of mine has been diagnosed with MS and another friend has been diagnosed with cancer. I'm the lucky one.'

So that was six years ago. And I've tried. I really have. In the first six months I lost quite a bit of weight. I tried to eat more healthily, which with my diet wouldn't have been difficult. Well, actually, it was very difficult and over the last six years I have yo-yoed in weight and found it incredibly difficult to stop eating all the things which exacerbate my diabetes. I felt a complete fraud when I was asked to be an ambassador for the charity Diabetes UK. They even featured me as their cover picture following an interview I did with them. Here's an excerpt from it:

'Having diabetes has never been an issue for Iain and after having classic symptoms for a couple of years, his diagnosis was hardly a shock. 'I was always thirsty and having to get up in the night to go to the loo, so when the GP told me I had diabetes, I wasn't at all surprised,' Iain recalls. 'She told me it shouldn't impact too much on my life if I made some lifestyle changes and took all the right medication, so I wasn't too concerned. Other people were more worried, but one of my friends was diagnosed with MS and another with cancer, so I count myself lucky.'

Although fifty-year-old Iain has lost two stone since his diagnosis, he admits there is still plenty of room for improvement. 'The worst thing the doctor said is that I should still be able to eat the things I like, as all the things I like are bad for me! I have got better. At one time I was drinking three litres of Fanta a day, but I have switched to mineral water and I love crisps but now I eat the baked variety.'

Iain thinks there are a lot of misconceptions about diabetes. He has written about it on his former blog, Iain Dale's Diary, which closed in July 2011, and he hopes to create a better understanding of the condition in a proposed new role as ambassador for Diabetes UK. Iain thinks people with diabetes need more positive support from the government. 'At the moment the approach is to lecture people into what might happen to them if they don't follow government advice, but I think it would be better to demonstrate the benefits of following a healthy lifestyle by giving people examples of how people have successfully controlled their diabetes.'

As far as practising what he preaches, and leading a healthy lifestyle goes, Iain tries to incorporate exercise into his daily routine, but is realistic about what he can achieve, given his hectic schedule. 'I used to play golf once a week but gave that up about two years ago. My life is so busy I find it hard to make the time, though in the summer I often hop on a Boris bike to ride the two miles between my publishing company and the LBC studios.' And — as far as eating food that is off limits goes — his philosophy is simple, 'It's OK to have a little of what you fancy — just don't eat the whole packet!'

Quick fire . . .

What three things would you abolish from a diabetes life?
A nagging partner, a nagging GP or nurse and blood tests! I have a dreadful sweet tooth and hate being told I can't have things and they can never find a vein and end up having to put the needle in the back of my hand.

What advice would you give to someone who has just been diagnosed with diabetes?
Don't think you're going to die and make changes

gradually. There can be a tendency for people to be a bit zealous when they are diagnosed, and to try and give everything up all at once. But people have to realise that this is a long-term condition and they have to change a little at a time.

Has diabetes brought anything positive to your life?
I would say that having diabetes has given me more knowledge about what I eat. I now look at the sugar, fat and carbohydrate content of the food I buy and have changed my diet quite a lot. I have lost about two stone since I was diagnosed and try and make healthy choices most of the time, then I go and spoil it all by eating a load of chocolate biscuits!

What's the strangest myth you have heard about diabetes?
I thought it was a joke when someone told me you were entitled to free Viagra on the NHS if you have diabetes, but then I found out it was true! I haven't had to use it yet, though.

What's the most and least healthy food in your fridge?
Melon and Leerdammer cheese.

I have a very, very sweet tooth. And I love carbs. I have tried so very hard to cut down, but I have tastes which don't often tally with healthy food. I'm not too keen on fish. I don't like salad. My only salvation is that I don't drink alcohol at all. At the time of writing, I haven't bought any chocolate for eight months or any sweets for six months. That's not to say I haven't eaten any, but not buying them has probably cut my consumption by 90 per cent. At one point I weighed close to nineteen stone. I now float between sixteen and a half and seventeen, which is still way above the recommended weight for my height of 6′2″.

I think I am quite typical for a diabetes sufferer. We try to block out from our minds that everything we eat that we shouldn't could result in losing our sight, having a limb amputated or having a stroke or heart attack far earlier than we otherwise could. It's the equivalent of sticking fingers in our ears and singing 'la la la, I can't hear you'.

And all this when the NHS provides free drugs for us. I'm on six pills a day at the moment, plus I now have to inject something called Victoza. It is not insulin, but it is supposed to reduce appetite.

But, of course, it's not all about diet, it ought to be about exercise too. But like a lot of other people I lead a busy life. I work unconventional hours. I have two jobs, which means I often work from 9 a.m. until 8 p.m. I skip breakfast so I can get an earlier train. I'll pop into M&S Food to get a sandwich for breakfast. On the odd occasion I forget to take my pills. I try not to do lunches with business or media contacts, but my lunch will also often consist of a sandwich, a packet of crisps and some fruit from Pret. Yes, fruit! I then don't eat until I get home at 9.30 p.m. at night. And there's no time for exercise in that schedule. I used to play tennis and squash. I gave them up in my thirties as I knew too many people older than that who'd had heart attacks on court. I have taken up golf again — the only sport I have ever been any good at — but it takes so much out of the day that I can only ever play at the weekend. I bought some running shoes, a cross trainer and a rowing machine. That happened a year ago. I haven't used them once.

So I'm as guilty as the next person in not taking responsibility for my own health. There are times I think that if I want to live to a ripe old age I should give up working in the media, move to Norfolk and do a normal nine-to-five job. But of course I won't. I love what I do too much.

All of this means that I, and many hundreds of thousands of people like me, cost the NHS a great deal more money than we ought to. There are now 3.8 million people living with diabetes in the UK and last year saw the biggest increase in new cases since 2008. In England alone, 768 people are diagnosed with Type 2 diabetes every day. The increase shows no signs of slowing down — five million people in the UK are projected to have diabetes by 2025. Left unchecked, the impact on the NHS and the nation's health will be immense.

Diabetes UK, in their paper titled 'The Cost of Diabetes', a report on an International Diabetes Federation study, shows that people with diabetes have medical costs that are two to three times more than age- and sex-matched patients without diabetes, i.e. that if the average healthcare cost per person is £1,000, for a similar person with diabetes it will be £2,000—£3,000.

Of course personal responsibility for one's health extends far beyond diet. For example, sexual health is something that many of us avoid thinking about because it's embarrassing. Who likes talking to their GP about yucky things like STDs. That's why STD clinics are so important. It's easy to be preachy and tell people they should behave, wear condoms and not take risks, but human beings err. They're not robots. This is one area where government policy over the years has worked in terms of educating people about risk. But I still wonder whether more resources ought to be put into GP training in this area and making clinics more accessible.

So, what to do? In the end, there's only a limited amount that the government can do. It can improve food labelling and information, so we all know what we are eating, and then make a judgement. It could incentivise food manufacturers to improve the healthiness of their products. Note that word 'incentivise'. In all aspects of health education and regulation there needs to be a lot more carrot and a lot less stick. The nanny state can only do so much to make us do things to improve our health. It should concentrate on encouraging us, rather than berating us.

9
Still the NHS Cinderella: mental health

Dealing with the challenges provided by mental health is possibly one of the most important challenges the NHS faces. It's become almost a cliché to describe mental health as a 'Cinderella service'. It's a subject too few people take seriously and one that some still find difficult to discuss. While the stigma of mental health has been eroded, it is still undoubtedly there.

When I started presenting on the radio four years ago, I never for one moment thought I would become known for my programmes on mental health, let alone be shortlisted for an award by the mental health charity MIND. But I can remember the heartbreaking calls I took when I first did a phone-in on depression. Frankly, I could have devoted this whole book to mental health and the problems associated with it.

Mental health covers a multitude of issues and when you look at the statistics on mental health, you wonder why more resources are not devoted to this area of health provision. One in four of us will suffer from some sort of mental health condition — not just in our lifetimes, but each year. And a quarter of those won't visit their GP. But the real question is what happens if they do visit their GPs? Anecdotal evidence from my listeners suggests that not enough GPs are equipped to deal with mental health issues. Maybe older GPs didn't have the same kind of mental health training which is available today, I don't know but, time after time, people tell me that their GPs seem out of their depth on these kinds of issues. And perhaps this explains why the prescription of drugs seems to be the automatic default for so many GPs.

But part of the problem is that people suffering from mental health problems, or their families, face a bewildering system which is so complex that even those who are familiar with it find it baffling. Okay, we have mental health trusts, but there are also acute trusts which provide liaison psychiatry services and some A&E services for mental health patients. Ambulance trusts may or may not be commissioned to provide mental health conveyancing services outside of emergencies, whatever they may be.

Clinical Commissioning Groups commission some services while Specialist Commissioning commissions others. And then, of course, there are GPs who provide primary mental health care to some 83 per cent of mental health patients. And then, finally, you have local authorities who oversee and/or directly employ Approved Mental Health Professionals — or at least those who are not employed by or seconded to the NHS.

I can't begin to cover all the aspects of mental health here, and I'm not going to try, but I do want to touch on dementia care. This is where the NHS and the social care system need to interact far better than they do at the moment. No one seems to have got to grips with the demands that the increasing number of people suffering from dementia are placing on both systems.

Everyone has good intentions but, so far, it has to be said that not a lot has changed recently. The trouble is that to provide a proper care system for people with dementia will mean that huge amounts of extra money needs to be spent, but where is it going to come from?

Indeed, the mental health budget is experiencing a 2 per cent cut. Beds continue to be closed and we are constantly told that it is far better to treat people in their homes. Really? The true heroes are the relatives who end up being carers for people with dementia. What we really need to do, even as a short-term fix, is to provide far better support for carers, especially more respite care. In effect, family carers are saving the NHS or the social care system hundreds of millions, if not several billion pounds, each year.

The Mental Health Action Plan which Nick Clegg announced was a welcome recognition that the current system isn't working, but it was really a list of aspirations rather than firm commitments. But things are moving in the right direction. It's great to see professional sports people be open about their mental health problems. It's great that politicians have publicly confronted their own issues surrounding their mental health. It's great that programmes like mine discuss this matter openly and without hesitation. None of those things would have happened ten years ago. If even just one person is helped by our discussions, and they realise they are not alone, I feel I have done something worthwhile.

10
Transparency and the right to know

The British Medical Association does a very good job, aided and abetted by the BBC, of making out it is a medical body. In fact, it is nothing of the sort. It is an aggressive trade union dedicated to fighting any sort of progressive reform in the health service. Switch on the *Today* programme of a morning and you'll inevitably find one of its representatives slagging off the government of the day for daring to do something which might be in the patients' interests rather than that of the doctors. Nowhere is this more apparent than in the area of a patient's right to know. The phrase 'sunshine is the best form of disinfectant' is one which has passed them by.

They fight every move to give the patient information about health outcomes or the performance of their local hospital. They say that individual statistics don't tell the whole story. They make out the statistics might be damaging to morale. In short, they always go out of their way to protect their vested interests. We shouldn't blame them or be surprised. That's what trade unions do. They don't exist to see the bigger picture. They exist to protect and promote the interests of their members. So when you hear a BMA representative explaining why the government is wrong, bear that in mind.

When health secretary Jeremy Hunt outlined plans to name GPs with a poor record of spotting cancer, the BMA was up in arms. Well, I don't know about you, but if my GP was poor at spotting cancer symptoms, I'd quite like to know about it. But no, according to the BMA it's the doctors' interests that must be protected at all costs. 'If you simply name and shame GPs, the tendency would be for us to refer everyone,' said Dr Chaand Nagpaul, the chairman of the BMA's GPs' committee. Just think about that for a moment. No one is suggesting 'naming and shaming' in that way that Dr Nagpaul implies. All the health secretary was doing was wanting to give patients more information. If Nagpaul's logic means anything, he is presumably against giving parents information about the performance of their child's school. He then issues the threat of referring everyone, just to be on the safe side, as if that would solve anything. It's typical of the BMA response to any suggestion that the patient might be empowered. I could cite their response to virtually any similar suggestion and it would be more or less identical. At times it's just best to ignore them because all they are interested in doing is protecting their vested interests. They complain the health secretary doesn't meet them very often. I'm not surprised. Perhaps he is waiting for them to have something valuable to say. It may be a long wait.

11
Diet and the nanny state

Another day, another front page story in the *Daily Express* about how something we like is damaging to us and the government is being urged to tax it. I have never understood why so-called health professionals appear to believe that the way to stop someone doing something which they consider is bad for them is to put an extra dollop of tax on it. Putting up the cost of a can of Fanta by 10p won't put a single person off drinking it. Adding 20p to a packet of chocolate digestives won't decrease our likelihood of eating them. So why do relatively intelligent people insist on proposing such things? Because it gets them in the media and makes them look important, is one cynical suggestion. But it must go deeper than that, surely.

It's the same 'nanny state' approach which leads otherwise perfectly rational politicians to seriously suggest that all cigarette packets should be wrapped in plain packaging. Apparently, we, the people, are less likely to buy them if they don't have any marketing images and blurb on the outside. Except that it's rubbish. This was tried in Australia and consumption actually rose.

So putting a tax on fizzy drinks isn't likely to do much good unless it is so prohibitive that we simply couldn't afford to buy them. And any such tax would, of course, be completely regressive and hit those at the bottom of the pile far harder than anyone else.

There's no doubt that our diet is a huge problem if we are to combat the mass onset of Type 2 diabetes. There's also little doubt as to what is causing this and it's our twenty-first-century society. But we can't punish people into changing their ways. We can't force people to eat vegetables rather than pre-packed vegetable samosas. If someone is told they must do something and it's for their own good, they aren't likely to receive it very well. All the people who adopt this approach need to take a course in basic psychology. We need more carrot and less stick. Indeed, we need to eat far more carrots than sticks of rock.

Let's take the recent government report

which recommends that sugar should only form 5 per cent of our daily energy intake, rather than the hitherto recommendation of 10 per cent. Well, on the face of it, it sounds eminently reasonable but, in reality, it is so unworkable as to render it useless as a recommendation. What it means is that if you drink one 330ml can of coke, you have already met your daily recommended sugar intake before you even eat anything else. As I say, totally impractical. The chief nutritionist at Public Health England then said: 'Instead of fizzy drinks have water or low-fat milk. Instead of a chocolate bar, have a piece of fruit.' On what planet do these people live? If it were that simple we'd all be doing it already.

The truth is that we will only change our diets when our lifestyles change. And I'm afraid that is going to take one hell of a long time. We all lead busy lives where processed foods have become part of our everyday diets. Fresh food is something we aspire to eat rather than eat every day. Processed foods take little preparation; they look nice and are relatively cheap. If two parents come home at 6 p.m., the last thing they want to do is spend two hours preparing a nutritious meal. No, they'll go to the freezer and put something in the microwave and feed the kids that way.

Of course consumer habits can be changed at the margins by government healthy eating campaigns but, in reality, the people the government need to attack are not the beleaguered consumers, it's the food manufacturers. It is they who need to reduce the sugar, salt and fat contents in a lot of their foods. Labelling is extremely important, but that is already very good. As a Type 2 diabetic, I know which fruit juices and drinks are the most dangerous for me because of the carbohydrate and sugar contents on the labels. Of course I shouldn't be drinking any sugary fruit juices, but if I allow myself the odd treat at least I know which product will do me least damage.

When I was first diagnosed, I thought I would have to give up everything I like, but soon came to realise that if I wanted to lose weight

I didn't actually have to give up eating all the things I really craved. If I picked and chose, I needn't just exist on rice and lentils. Take crisps, as an example. I love crisps. Always have. Always will. But by looking at the labels on the packets, I can reduce my fat and carbohydrate content massively if I choose a packet of Walkers Baked crisps rather than a packet of McCoys. But that's only because I have acquired the knowledge to know what to look for. How many normal people pick up every single product and look at the fat content or carbs content? Very few, I suggest.

Conclusion

Let me give you some predictions. First, all politicians will tell you that the NHS is their number-one priority. The NHS has achieved the same status as the Queen Mother in the nation's affections.

But I do not see an appetite to change it fundamentally and, as a consequence, I think over time it will become a much hotter political potato than it may be at the moment; as expectations increase, performance will lag behind.

The challenge facing all politicians will be how to square this unsquareable circle. The truth is that they will abdicate responsibility to health professionals and then blame them if it all goes wrong.

In future, most government initiatives are likely to be centred around preventative measures rather than structural ones. Preventative healthcare has grown in visibility in recent times. An anti-obesity drive is always guaranteed to provoke big headlines in the mid-market newspapers as well as intense discussion on radio phone-ins.

Such initiatives give the appearance of action, even if they can be incredibly expensive in PR costs. Politicians love them. They are great for photo opportunities, sound bites and gimmickry. So expect a lot more of junior health ministers exhorting us in their best nanny-like tones to eat less, drink less and exercise more. I think I need a lie-down.

There needs to be a national and rational debate about the scope and extent of the NHS. Should it cover illness, injuries or both? Should people insure against injury — probably a small cost — as opposed to illness? But I pity the first politician to even suggest such heresy.

Can we afford to maintain the 'cradle to grave' scope that Beveridge established? Having asked that, I doubt that he foresaw the range of treatments currently available and their cost. I doubt also that he foresaw a health service where 2,600 people earn more than the prime minister, and 7,800 people earn more than £100,000 a year.

The bald truth is that until we accept that the NHS can't and never will be able to meet all the demands made on it, we can't actually have a proper and rational debate.

The pity is that no one currently on the NHS scene seems to have much idea of the questions, let alone the answers. Parliaments drift by and the issues and questions remain the same: expensive reorganisations take place with little or no real benefit. And anyone who dares to criticise or critique the NHS gets their head bitten off by people who profess to LOVE the NHS.

So the real, overwhelming question is this: if we were in a position to set up a health service now, from scratch, what would it look like? Because I suspect one thing is certain — it would bear little relation to the NHS we have today.

50 things which could make the NHS better

1. We need to have a prolonged national debate about the future of healthcare provision
2. Health secretaries should be left in post for longer
3. Scrap national pay bargaining
4. Improve procurement procedures and price bargaining
5. Embrace private sector involvement where it leads to higher standards and lower cost
6. Politicians must stop trying to frighten people that the NHS is about to be privatised — private sector involvement is very different to privatisation
7. The private sector can provide extra capacity when the NHS lacks it
8. The NHS should cease being so defensive about legitimate criticism
9. Charges for GP visits should be considered
10. Charging people for A&E treatment when they have been negligent (drunks, for example)
11. No foreign visitor should be treated without producing insurance papers. In all other circumstances, charges must be levied
12. The NHS should no longer fund most cosmetic surgery, tattoo removal or gastric band operations

13. Accept that the profit motive is not anathema in healthcare

14. End the system where if people pay for private treatment, the NHS then refuses to offer any further treatment

15. Employers should be incentivised to provide healthcare for their staff

16. The NHS should accept the localism agenda

17. Hospitals operating theatres should be utilised seven days a week, not five, to ensure patient safety and quality of service no matter what time of day or day of the week you go into hospital

18. Put the cost of each drug on the label

19. Care for the elderly needs to be radically overhauled

20. Recognise that small can be beautiful in the NHS. It's not all about large general hospitals. Cottage hospitals and specialist units need to thrive and not be undermined

21. There should be tax breaks for families who act as carers

22. There should be compulsory insurance to pay for care in old age

23. There should be top-up payments for some treatments

24. There should be less 'nanny state', less stick and more carrot

25. Personal responsibility for our health is something the state should put more emphasis on in health education campaigns

26. A major effort to improve cancer survival should be launched

27. The Cancer Drugs Fund needs to be reformed and given more power

28. GP surgeries need to open at times when working people are able to use them

29. There must be more local accountability for the way the NHS performs

30. Consultation processes need to be improved so people can have confidence in them

31. Nursing training needs to be re-examined, especially entry-level qualifications which are far too onerous

32. We need to stop recruiting so many foreign nurses and doctors and look at training more in this country

33. Dementia care needs to be improved dramatically, with the pressure being taken off charities

34. Generic drugs should be used more often, to replace more expensive branded drugs

35. The prescription system needs to be changed to reward personal responsibility. For example, diabetes patients should be required to pay for their prescriptions if they don't meet blood sugar targets set by their GPs

36. Erectile dysfunction drugs, like Viagra, should no longer be available as a free prescription (which it currently is for diabetes patients if they ask for it)

37. Car parking charges should be scrapped, with the £200 million cost met through improved procurement processes

38. An inquiry needs to be held into the salaries of top executives in the NHS

39. As part of David Cameron's EU renegotiations, he should exempt healthcare from the 48-Hour Working Week Directive

40. Nurses should, where possible, work on the same wards each week to provide continuity of care

41. Nurses and doctors should be expected to speak excellent English, *especially* those on geriatric wards

42. The two main political parties need to agree the way ahead on social care

43. It must be recognised that the NHS can't fund every new drug and every new treatment

44. Priority must be given to keeping the diabetes budget under control

45. GPs need better training in diagnosing depression and other forms of mental illness

46. Mental health policy needs a Royal Commission

47. Taxing unhealthy drinks and food won't work in any meaningful way

48. Hospital cleanliness needs to be improved. Chief executives need to be held directly accountable for failures in cleanliness, with 20 per cent of their salary being withheld for repeat offences

49. Sexual health needs more resourcing

50. Managers fired for incompetence or maladministration, or who receive large pay-offs, should never again be employed by the NHS

About LBC

LBC is Britain's only national news talk radio station. It tackles the big issues of the day, with intelligent, informed and provocative opinion from guests, listeners and presenters, including Nick Ferrari, James O'Brien, Shelagh Fogarty, Iain Dale, Ken Livingstone, David Mellor and Beverley Turner. LBC reaches 1.2 million people in Britain and is available on DAB digital radio, online at lbc.co.uk, through mobile apps, Sky Digital Channel 0112, Virgin Media Channel 919 and on 97.3FM in London.

About the Series

In this major new series, popular LBC presenters tackle the big issues in politics, current affairs and society. We might applaud their views; we might be outraged. But these short, sharp polemics are destined to generate controversy, discussion and debate — and lead Britain's conversation.

Titles in the series

Steve Allen, *So You Want to Be a Celebrity?*

Duncan Barkes, *The Dumbing Down of Britain*

Iain Dale, *The NHS: Things That Need to Be Said*

Nick Ferrari, *It's Politics ... But Not As We Know It*

James O'Brien, *Loathe Thy Neighbour*